RELAX
YOUR MIND

*SIMPLE MEDITATION
TECHNIQUES TO RELIEVE
STRESS AND QUIET A BUSY
MIND*

THOMAS CALABRIS

Check out our website at:
www.EliminateStressNow.com

Relax Your Mind
Publisher : Inner Vitality Systems, LLC.
Website : www.EliminateStressNow.com
ISBN : 978-1-7329106-0-7

Disclaimer

The Information presented in this publication is intended as an educational resource and is not intended as a substitute for proper medical advice. All readers are encouraged to seek proper professional and medical advice when needed. This book is not for anyone that has medical mental conditions. Do not read this book and seek proper medical treatment if you have serious mental illness.

The author and publisher of this material are not responsible in any manner whatsoever for any action or injury which may occur by reading or following the instruction in this document. The author cannot be held responsible for any personal or commercial damage caused by misinterpretation of the information or improper use of the information.

No patent liability is assumed with respect to the use of the information contained herein. Although every precaution has been taken in the preparation of this book, the publisher and author assume no responsibility for errors or omissions.

WHY I WROTE THIS BOOK

I have studied various forms of meditation for almost thirty years. My teachers have inspired me to strive to live a healthy and empowered life. I have benefited tremendously from the knowledge and wisdom they have taught me.

One of the most important lessons I have learned is that of service. That is being of service to others. When we support each other and focus our mind-power on a common goal, the power is amplified and everyone benefits.

So now it is time for me to be of service to others. And the best way I know to be of service to others is by sharing my love of meditation and other forms of natural health solutions with others. Thus, I wrote this book with the hope of passing on the knowledge and experience I have gained from my teachers to others.

WHY YOU SHOULD READ THIS BOOK

There are many benefits of practicing meditation, including stress relief. The techniques taught in this book have been around for centuries. More recently, modern research and studies have shown the true benefits of meditation like inducing a relaxation response, reducing blood pressure, and much more.

There is an epidemic of stress in the world. The effects of stress are very costly, both in terms of the toll on the body and the mind and in terms of monetary cost. Health care costs are higher than ever.

This book is for those people looking for a natural approach to relieving stress and calming their minds. This book will give you a step-by-step approach to stress relief and relaxing your mind through meditation. I have personally benefited from the meditation techniques taught in this book and you can benefit from them too.

If you are looking for a natural and cost-effective solution for reducing the effects of stress, improving your health, and achieving inner peace, then this book is for you. While meditation is not meant to replace traditional health care, meditation can complement it and provide a foundation for healing.

TABLE OF CONTENTS

PREFACE

"Magic is believing in yourself, if you can do that, you can make anything happen."
- Goethe

It is often assumed that a person that has practiced meditation for many years must never get stressed out. This couldn't be further from the truth. While I have practiced various forms of meditation for almost thirty years, I still live in the same world as everyone else and face the same issues in life that everyone else faces.

While meditation is one of my passions, I still have a day job as a software engineer, which I have worked at for over twenty years. It is a stressful job that comes with a lot of responsibilities. I have at times let the job take over my life and let the stress affect my health negatively. However, it is because of my study of meditation and other natural forms of healing that I am able to bring myself back into balance.

Stress causes imbalances in both the mind and the body. Living a life of balance means that you balance both your mind and your body. When you are in balance, it will be easy to relax your mind and body. The meditation practices taught in this book will help to bring balance back to your mind and body. You will learn valuable techniques that can be applied at any stage of your life, easy or difficult, to *"relax your mind"*.

It is important to practice these techniques daily when life is easy, so that you will know what to do when life is more difficult. It is my hope that you will learn and practice these meditation techniques and you too will benefit as I have.

CHAPTER 1 – INTRODUCTION

"You don't have to see the whole staircase, just take the first step."
- Martin Luther King Jr.

Have you ever wanted to sleep but your mind kept racing with the thoughts of the day? Have you ever tried to focus on something, like reading, but you couldn't concentrate because thoughts of what needed to be done wouldn't stop? *I need to pick up the kids from school. What should I cook for dinner? My boss is constantly on my case for no reason. Why can't I lose weight?*

At times, it can be difficult to quiet our minds, especially when we are under a lot of stress. Constant worrying trains our subconscious or autonomic nervous system, our subconscious mind, to automatically repeat the types of thoughts that we *"feed"* it.

It is often said that in today's world, we are more *"human doing"* than *"human being"*. There is so much to do and so little time. And with all of our electronic communications, like cell phones and computers, we are in constant contact with people, news, and other sound bites of information.

Thus, it seems difficult at times to shut things down and experience peace and quiet. It literally leads to an addiction. There is now a medical term for people that experience anxiety when they can't access their mobile technology; it is called Nomophobia. [1]

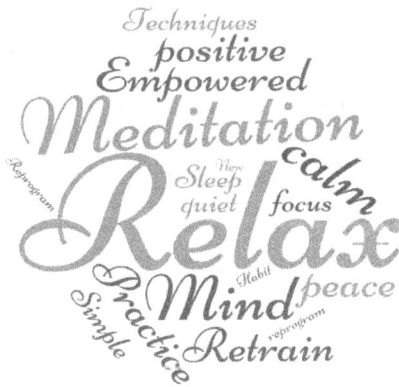

So how can we quiet our minds and prevent these negative automatic or subconscious thoughts from taking over? I propose that we can do this through meditation. While the benefits of meditation have been known for centuries, there has been a lot of research recently that has shed new light on the benefits of meditation.

While relaxation is one of the obvious benefits of meditation, a recent study has shown that the brain structure is actually changed, for the better. For eight weeks of meditation practice of 30 minutes per day, meditation was shown to cause the brain to increase the density of Grey matter (neurons) in areas important for learning and memory. [2]

Several other studies showed that mindfulness meditation significantly improved or reduced anxiety, stress, and depression. [3] Also, it was found that mindfulness meditation was moderately successful at alleviating pain, anxiety, depression, and improving the quality of sleep. [4][5]

In the coming chapters, I will explain what stress is and how it affects your body and mind. I will show you simple meditation techniques to reduce stress and to reduce or eliminate negative programmed thoughts, to relax and retrain the mind.

Simply put, I will show you easy to follow steps to relax your mind and to transform not only your mind, but your way of being. All that I ask is that you have an open mind and practice these techniques daily and consistently to get the benefits.

These are the same techniques that I have learned from my teachers, in various healing traditions, over the years and have used them in my own life to relax and retrain my mind. It is easy in life to find yourself going down a stressful path. Encountering something outside of our comfort zone is part of the human experience. However, it is our perceptions and courage to take action that determines if we stay and live in the stress.

These are the techniques that I choose to return to especially when I have been taken down one of those stressful paths and find myself stressed and out of balance. So I take action with these techniques to keep myself from being stuck in stress and fear and to transform them into stepping stones for an empowered life. The key take away message for you is that it is up to you to make a choice and take action to restore your balance and relax your mind.

At the end of each chapter, you will find a section called *"Action Steps"*. These *"Action Steps"* are the steps you need to take to put into action the information provided in the chapter. It is only when you take action that you will change your habits and begin to reduce your stress.

It is often said that it takes twenty-one days to form a new habit. So I invite you to practice the techniques presented here for twenty-one days. Make eliminating stress a habit in your life. And it starts now with the next chapter.

CHAPTER 2 – STRESS AFFECTS THE BODY AND THE MIND

"Stress is caused by being 'here' but wanting to be 'there'."
- Eckhart Tolle

Research shows that between 75% and 90% of all doctor's visits are due to stress [6]. This means that stress is at epidemic levels. In this chapter, we will look at what stress is and how it affects both the body and the mind.

First, what exactly is stress? Stress is a physiological response to a perception that something is going to harm you (the stressor), whether it is real or imagined. This response, called fight or flight, is characterized by the activation of the sympathetic nervous system, which prepares the body (biochemically) to handle the stress [7].

During a stressful event (real or imagined), the adrenal glands produce chemicals or hormones like adrenaline, nor-epinephrine, and cortisol. Adrenaline increases your heart rate. Nor-epinephrine redirects blood flow to bodily functions necessary for handling stress like muscles. Cortisol maintains blood pressure, regulates the bodily functions necessary to handle the stress and suppresses those functions that are not important for the stress at hand. This is important if you need to get out of the way of an oncoming car as you cross the street. Thus, for real physical stress, it is a good thing. It is often-times the imagined stress that gets us into trouble and can lead to chronic stress.

Long-term stress becomes chronic and the stress-induced chemicals take a toll on the body and the mind. Cortisol kills neurons of the brain that are responsible for memory. Over time, the adrenals may become weakened or fatigued, which can leave you feeling exhausted. A constant increased heart rate can lead to high blood pressure if left unchecked.

A person under chronic stress can develop a nervous system that is dominated by the sympathetic nervous system. This means that a person is living with active stress pathways in their nervous system. They are living close to fight or flight. They are living with tension in the body and generating inflammation. Also, the immune system is suppressed.

Thus, physically, chronic stress negatively affects digestion, immune function, detoxification, concentration, memory, and increased blood pressure, to name a few, all of which may lead to one or more health issues. And mentally, chronic stress can also cause anxiety, depression, irritability, and a feeling of being overwhelmed, to name a few symptoms.

As I have mentioned previously, during stressful events, the sympathetic nervous system dominates and the parasympathetic nervous system is suppressed. The parasympathetic nervous system is responsible for healing, growth, repairing, detoxification, and cleaning the body.

Now that we know what stress is, what can we do to relieve the effects of stress? Or better yet, what can we do to reduce or eliminate stress itself? It is important to point out that when we relax both the body and the mind, we can achieve a state called, *"The Relaxation Response"*, where the parasympathetic nervous system is activated [8].

It is during this *"relaxation response"* that we begin the process of healing from the effects of stress. Thus, it is imperative that we learn to recognize the true cause of the chronic stress so we can properly deal with it.

While chronic stress triggers vary from person-to-person, the underlying cause is always the same. The underlying cause of stress is fear. Fear is an emotional reaction to our perception that something will harm us in some way or cause us pain.

In times of danger, this is a good thing to motivate us, like running away from a wild animal. But in today's world, we can feel threatened by things that are not likely to harm us, but we perceive that they will. Once in a while, this will not cause us any issues. However, if self-induced stress becomes a daily occurrence, then it can begin to affect our health as we discussed previously.

It is important to examine the root cause of your stress and your fears. Often-times, we try to numb ourselves to avoid the emotional pain that we feel. This only compounds the issue. In the next chapter, we will learn that the first step to recognizing our fears is to live in the *"here and now"*.

Action Steps

It is now time to awaken your consciousness and take action. Take a look at your stress. What fear(s) are the root cause of your stress? You may have to dig deep. If you are stuck, ask a trusted friend or spouse what triggers your stress. They may surprise you with their answer. Start a journal. Be honest with yourself and write them down. Once you become aware of your fears, you can take steps to eliminate them.

CHAPTER 3 – HERE AND NOW

"If you are depressed, you live in the past...
If you are anxious, you live in the future...
But, if you are at peace... You live in the
present."
- Lao Tzu

We can learn to reduce stress and fear by living in the present moment, the **"here and now"**. The present moment is all we really ever have. We must learn from and accept the past. But it is over. The past is history and it can't be changed. So let it go. Don't let the past direct your life. Don't let it keep you from living in the present moment.

All it takes for you to be in the *"here and now"* or the present moment is for you to make a choice. Make a choice to live in the present moment. It is difficult because we have conditioned our minds to constantly race and worry about the past and the future. *"I was hurt by so and so..."* or *"What will they think of me?"* or *"What if they don't like me?"* It can be about traumatic events. It can also be about mundane everyday things. But our minds are always racing.

We can overcome this overactive mind. Over time, our subconscious mind becomes programmed with these racing thoughts and eventually we do it without thinking or subconsciously.

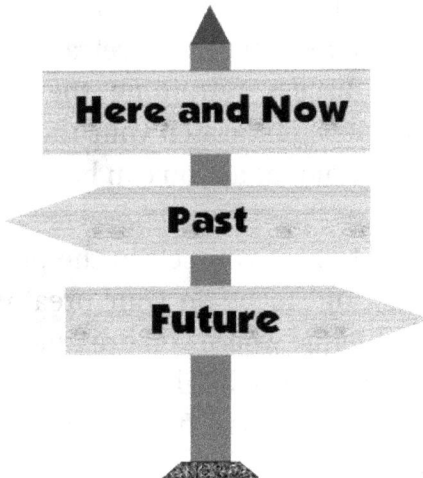

Which one do you choose?

But it will take conscious effort and practice to reprogram or retrain our subconscious mind, which will free our conscious mind. Don't you want conscious control over your thoughts instead of having your subconscious mind playing these random negative thoughts over and over? I do and I'll bet you do too.

The retraining of the mind begins with *"silent witnessing"*. Just be aware of the things that you think about without judging yourself. Silently witness your thoughts, feelings, and actions. Notice how you are feeling in any moment, especially fearful or stressful moments. Notice what is triggering you to feel that way.

It is very important that you don't judge yourself. No judgments. Just the conscious awareness or *"witnessing"* has the potential to retrain our minds over time. We will discuss retraining the mind more in Chapter 6. For now, just watch your thoughts and be as present in each moment as you can be.

Another way to root yourself in the present moment is to sit quietly and focus on your breathing. This is a meditation technique where you breathe deeply into the abdomen with each breath. Then you count your breath cycles. Inhale, exhale, 1. Inhale, exhale, 2. Inhale, exhale, 3. Continue to count your breath for a minute or as long as you want.

Sitting in silence and just being a **"silent witness"** to your thoughts is a type of meditation. In the following chapters, you will be introduced to additional meditation techniques to help relax your mind, like repeating a mantra or positive affirmation, abdominal breathing, visualization, and more.

Forgiveness and gratitude are important keys to living in the present moment. Let's first start with forgiveness. Forgive those that have harmed you verbally or physically. It doesn't mean you should condone their actions, but you can forgive them and let it go so you can move on.

Holding on to grudges only keeps you stuck in the past. As Nelson Mandela said, *"Resentment is like drinking poison and then hoping it will kill your enemies."* It never works. So what are you still holding on to from your past? It is time to take an inventory of the things you are holding on to from your past. Be honest with yourself.

When living in the present moment, it is also important to recognize and be grateful for your life. What are you grateful for? How about the fact that you can breathe? How about having a loving family and friends? How about that you have been given the opportunity to take this journey we call life? There are so many things to be grateful for. It is difficult to feel stress when you in a state of gratitude.

I recommend starting a gratitude journal. Every day find five new things that you are grateful for and write them down. It is so simple, but it is very powerful. Then when you feel like you are going down a stressful path, you can review your gratitude journal and remind yourself how wonderful life really is. Letting go of fear and feeling gratitude are the gateways to relaxing the mind. We go over "relaxing the mind" in the next chapter.

Action Steps

It is time to root yourself in the present moment. Start by taking action by doing *"silent witnessing"*. Watch yourself during the day. Without judgment, notice when you are not in the present moment. Notice when you are thinking about the past and the future. Write what you are noticing in your journal. What are your fear and stress triggers? It may surprise you. Also, write down five things you are grateful for and feel the gratitude in your heart. Things (stress, anxiety, fear) are now beginning to shift and change. Can you feel the weight of stress starting to lift?

CHAPTER 4 – RELAXING THE MIND

"Tension is who you think you should be.
Relaxation is who you are."
- Chinese Proverb

Usually when someone talks about relaxing, they are referring to relaxing the body. However, I have found that the body relaxes more quickly and deeply if the mind is relaxed. That is why relaxing the mind is very important. So you may be asking, "What do you mean by relaxing the mind?"

As I have said previously, people are constantly busy and living with stress in their daily lives. They are watching the kids, working, constantly checking their cellphones, email, Twitter, and Facebook, to name a few. We have an epidemic of texting while driving. I often see families walking in the park and at least one member is talking on the cellphone.

Our minds are constantly racing, thinking about where we have been and where we are going. More typically, the thoughts we have are negative and worrisome. Research has shown that on average, a person talks (thoughts) to themselves 50,000 times per day. 80% of these thoughts are negative. [9]

As a result, it is no wonder that we have a difficult time trying to quiet our minds. So when we talk about relaxing the mind, we mean to let go of all the mental chatter and to quiet the mind.

Have you ever gone to bed, feeling very tired, but you just can't seem to sleep? It's like every thought we've ever had comes rushing into our minds. It is very frustrating when you can't sleep because your mind is racing. I think we can all relate to this. It has happened to me on occasion. And now that I know how to relax my mind, it doesn't keep me up in bed at night.

There are several stages that you will go through to relax your mind. The stages are: focusing the mind, quieting the mind, and then finally retraining the mind. We will cover focusing the mind and quieting the mind in this chapter. In chapter 6, we will cover retraining the mind.

You can focus the mind when it is racing by concentrating on one thing. You could just count numbers. You could just repeat a word. Or you could repeat a positive affirmation or a mantra. I personally find repeating a positive affirmation to be most effective for me.

Here are some examples of positive affirmations:

1. I am calm, peaceful, and relaxed.

2. I am grateful for all the abundance in my life.

3. I am happy.

4. I am energized.

5. I love my life.

You get the idea. To be most effective, choose a positive affirmation that addresses your worry or stress. Don't make it too long or complicated. Once you have chosen your positive affirmation, find a quiet place where you won't be interrupted. Set aside five to ten minutes to simply relax.

Sit in a comfortable position and close your eyes. Take several deep breaths and be in the present moment. Now slowly repeat your positive affirmation constantly for the entire time. If you find that you are distracted by some thoughts, don't force things and don't get frustrated. Just return your focus to repeating your affirmation. Your mind will learn to better focus with practice. If you find your mind racing after you get into bed, you can use this technique to focus and relax your mind. Repeat, *"I am now getting sleepier and sleepier."* or *"I am ready for a good night's sleep."* Be creative.

Research has shown many benefits to repeating positive affirmations. Using positive affirmations can rewire the brain's neurons (neuroplasticity) to increase the connections in the brain for more positive thoughts and feelings. [10] Other research has shown that using positive affirmations can help improve self-esteem, depression, and other mental health issues. [11]

Once you have mastered focusing your mind (will take some time), then you can try to simply quiet your mind. Try to eliminate your thoughts all together. Don't think anything. It is easy to say and difficult to do.

If you find it too difficult, then just go back to repeating your positive affirmation. However, this time, put your attention on the silence or the spaces between the words. For *"I am relaxed"*, focus on the space between the words. Practice the following, *"I"* (pause for a few seconds) *"am"* (pause for a few seconds) *"relaxed"*. Just be present in the spaces.

This is a simple technique for learning to focus on the nothingness or the space between the words. You will get better with consistent practice. Consistent practice is the key to learning how to relax your mind. Don't expect to be perfect, just be consistent with your daily practice.

Action Steps

Take time now to create your own **positive affirmation** or use one of the above affirmations. Keep it simple and positive. Write your affirmation down in your journal. Now focus your mind by repeating your affirmation in the manner described in this chapter for five to ten minutes.

When you are done, write in your journal about your experience. How did you feel? Was it easy or difficult? Be honest. As you continue to practice this daily, you will notice that it gets easier to focus your mind.

CHAPTER 5 – ABDOMINAL BREATHING

"If you want to conquer the anxiety of life, live in the moment, live in the breath. "
- Chinese Proverb

If you are stressed, it is likely that you are breathing shallowly and therefore, you are not getting adequate amounts of oxygen and energy. Your body may become acidic. You may have an increased heart rate and even high blood pressure. The good news is that all of these can be avoided or reversed with proper abdominal breathing.

Abdominal breathing is another meditation technique to help relax your mind. Focusing on your breathing is a way to focus your mind's attention, taking it off the chatter and worry and being in the present moment with your breathing.

Unlike chest or shallow breathing, breathing into your abdomen allows your lungs to fill up optimally, thus increasing the amount of oxygen and energy that we can absorb and circulate. Then, you will exhale more carbon dioxide, which is acidic to the blood stream, thus, helping to balance the blood's pH (measure of acid/alkaline concentration). It is not only relaxing, but it is also energizing.

I recommend finding a place where you won't be interrupted. Sit in a comfortable position and close your eyes. As you inhale through your nose, allow your abdomen to gently and slowly expand. And when you exhale through your nose, allow your abdomen to gently and slowly move inward.

The characteristics of proper abdominal breathing are: **slow, long, thin, even, and soft**. Do not try to force your breathing. Just let it come naturally. If you get distracted by your thoughts, just notice them and let them go and return to your breathing.

In the beginning if you find it difficult to breathe into your abdomen, you can place your hands on your navel. Then as you inhale, your hands should move outward. And when you exhale, your hands should move inward.

Another technique is to lie down on a bed and place a book on your navel. As you inhale, the book should move up as your abdomen expands. And as you exhale the book should move down. Give it a try.

There are many benefits to abdominal breathing. Here are some benefits.

Increased Oxygen Intake During Inhalation

Increased oxygen intake enhances oxygen circulation to cells around the body. This facilitates energy production, healing due to disease and injury, and repairing due to normal wear and tear on the body. By expanding the abdomen during inhalation, this allows the lungs to fill up with air more completely. Regular breathing in this manner prevents so called "dead spaces" to occur in the lungs where little to no oxygen (O_2) and carbon dioxide (CO_2) is exchanged due to inadequate ventilation, which may lead to the collapse of the alveoli (small sacs where oxygen exchange takes place with blood vessels inside the lungs). Abdominal breathing can prevent these collapses by enhancing the production of surfactant. Surfactant is a compound produced in the wall of active alveolar sac that prevents the sac walls from sticking together. Thus, adequate breathing plays such an important role in your health. [12]

Increased Carbon Dioxide (CO_2) Release Through Exhalation

In physiology, there are complex mechanisms that occur in the body to balance the pH or acidity and alkalinity. Respiration or breathing is one of these mechanisms. When we exhale through the lungs, we expel among other things, CO_2, which is acidic. Thus, exhaling is a major way in which we release acid from the blood and body. People that are shallow breathers tend to be more acidic and there can be long term consequences (respiratory acidosis). The body then has to try to compensate in other ways to get rid of the acidic build up. Of course the opposite is also true, if you breathe too quickly, like hyperventilating, then you can get rid of too much CO_2 and the body can become too alkaline. That is why we were told to breathe into a paper bag if we hyperventilate. We are then inhaling the CO_2 captured in the bag that we got rid of too quickly. Thus, slow abdominal breathing helps to bring balance to many aspects of our physiology, including pH. [12]

Absorb More Energy While Breathing

As we breathe, we absorb energy (also known as Qi, pronounced chee) from our surroundings. This energy is stored in the energy centers of the body until it is needed. This is a fundamental concept of Traditional Chinese Medicine and Qigong, pronounced chee gung. Abdominal breathing allows us to take in more energy than we take in during normal and shallow breathing.

Reduced Heart Rate and Blood Pressure

Abdominal breathing reduces the heart rate and blood pressure, both of which reduces the demands on the heart. Slower abdominal breathing calms and relaxes the body. This is picked up by the autonomic nervous system to reduce the heart rate and blood pressure.

Calms and Relaxes the Body

When your mind is focused on abdominal breathing, it relaxes and lets go of other thoughts, thus reducing the effects of stress. This allows the autonomic nervous system to enter a state of parasympathetic dominance, which allows the body to repair and heal. It also allows for better digestion, circulation, and immune function.

Massages the Internal Organs

The mechanical motion of abdominal breathing actually massages the organs. This helps to increase the circulation of both energy and oxygen in the organs. Thus, improving the circulation in the organs allows the organs and the body to work more efficiently and effectively. If the energy is stagnant in your organs when you begin the abdominal breathing practice, you may notice improvements in your health with every day of practice. Consistent daily practice will yield the best results.

There are a lot of opportunities to practice abdominal breathing in our daily lives. You can do abdominal breathing while standing in line at the grocery store, while waiting in the doctor's office, while riding on the bus, while sitting at your desk, and many other situations. Be creative. The more you practice the better you will get at it and the benefits will follow. So practice, practice, practice.

Action Steps

Take time now to practice abdominal breathing. Find a comfortable place. Sit down, close your eyes, and be in the present moment with your abdominal breathing. Practice for between two to five minutes to start.

When you are done, write in your journal and describe your experience. How did you feel? Practice daily to get the most benefits. Schedule time to practice and make it a part of your daily life.

CHAPTER 6 – RETRAINING THE MIND

"The secret to change is to focus all of your energy not into fighting the old but on building the new."
- Chinese Proverb

Actually, at this point, if you've been practicing relaxing your mind and doing abdominal breathing, then you are already on your way to retraining your mind. When I talk about retraining, I mean to stop the negative thoughts from beginning in the first place.

As I have said previously, the worry and stress come about because we are having fearful thoughts. So while focusing your mind is an important first step, it is important to address the root cause of your fears and let them go for optimal relaxation of the mind.

Here are some tips for handling your fears.

1. Begin to recognize that you don't have to be perfect. No one is.

2. Living in the present moment, not the past or future, is the key to eliminating fears.

3. Identify your fear(s) and create a positive affirmation that positively addresses the fear(s). Repeat this affirmation as many times during the day as possible.

4. Talk your fears out with a good friend or a mentor. Sometimes explaining our fears to others helps us to realize how unnecessary the fears are.

5. Have faith in yourself that you can handle the situation without being fearful.

Change is often a big source of our fears. We like the consistency, the *"sure thing"* or *"what we've always done"*. There tends to be a lot of uncertainty associated with our thoughts about change. There is a lot of fear around our perceptions of this uncertainty. So it is now time to change our perceptions about *"change"* itself.

Change usually comes in two parts. First, there is the ending of something. Then there is the new or different thing that emerges (a new beginning). It is sometimes hard for us to let go of something that we are so familiar and comfortable with, even if it makes our lives miserable. This happens because we have been subconsciously programmed to react in this way.

It is sometimes hard to say goodbye to things and people. We fear being along. We fear that if we let go of a bad job, we may not get another one. Over time, these fears and our reaction to these fears become programmed in our subconscious mind. Then we have feelings and react to situations without even a conscious thought.

Sometimes our fears are over that new thing that might happen in the future. I won't find another job or I won't find a better girlfriend or boyfriend. With fear, it is always our perception about a situation that needs to change.

I hope you are seeing how these fears and negative perceptions, which are actually conscious thoughts, program our subconscious mind when they are repeated with strong emotions. They become imprinted on the subconscious mind, which is nothing more than strong neural pathways constructed in the autonomic nervous system of our brain.

They are physical constructs that have resulted from our conscious thoughts. These are the very pathways that we want to change or retrain. We do this by taking our attention off what we don't want consciously, and putting our attention on what we do want consciously.

Life is always going to be full of uncertainty and change. But our perceptions about change do not need to be one of negativity and resistance. We must look at change as new possibilities or opportunities. We must remain open minded. This requires a level of faith in ourselves. Can you have faith in yourself amidst the uncertainties of life?

So how do we change our perceptions and develop a profound faith in ourselves, so that when change and uncertainty come that we handle it in a more beneficial way? We can learn to trust in our intuition or our "gut feelings". We can also feed our minds with positive and beneficial thoughts and actions daily.

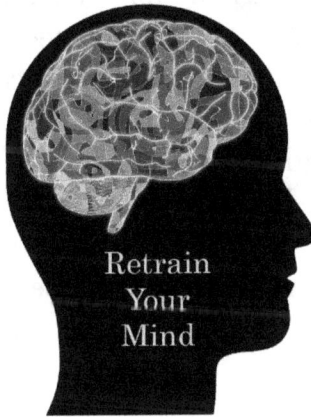

Retrain
Your
Mind

Change your self-talk. You have a choice as to what you think about. If a negative thought comes to your mind (old pattern), observe it but don't resist it. If you resist it then you just give more energy to the negative thought, thus re-enforcing it. Then think something positive or repeat an appropriate affirmation or mantra several times. It is the act of conscious choice and repetition that are your tools to retrain your mind.

Another tool to retrain your mind is visualization. In the next chapter, you will learn about the power of visualization and how you can use it to retrain your mind.

Action Steps

Take out your journal and write down your biggest fears. What is the driving force behind your fears? Is it because you don't want to be judged? Is it because you don't trust yourself? There are many causes of our fears.

Be honest with yourself and write them down. You can't reduce or eliminate your fears if you aren't aware of the causes. For each fear, write down a positive way to deal with your fear. It may be as simple as just changing your thoughts to be positive about the "fearful" situation.

CHAPTER 7 – VISUALIZATION

"Look within!... The secret is inside you."
- Hui-neng

Visualization is one of the most powerful techniques for retraining your mind. Your mind can't tell the difference between that which is real and that which is imagined or visualized. So it is important that when you visualize, you keep it positive and empowering.

Athletes have been known to use visualization to improve their performance, to perfect a golf swing or to perfect a foul shot or to improve one's speed. It has been used by Arnold Schwarzenegger for weightlifting, Billie Jean King for tennis, Lindsey Von of the U.S. Women's Olympics Ski Team, and many others. So why isn't this mainstream for everyday living or reducing or eliminating stress or healing?

Actually, it is an ancient technique that is regaining attention in our modern times. Visualization has been used for thousands of years in Eastern cultures for health and wellness. It is an important part of Qigong meditation practices, for instance, to assist with moving energy within the body for healing. Qigong is a combination of exercises, meditations, and breathing forms that originated in China around 5000 years ago.

Visualization can be used for just about any situation. It's effectiveness is only limited by your own imagination. You can visualize by seeing a desired situation in your mind's eye. Imagine that all of your five senses are involved. See the sights, hear the sound, feel the feelings. Leave nothing out. The more vivid the situation, the more impact it will have on your mind, especially your subconscious mind that you are trying to retrain.

For example, if you want to relax, see yourself in a calm situation, such as in a hot tub, or in nature, or anywhere that you feel comfortable and relaxed. Feel the warmth of the water on your body. Hear the jets moving and swirling the water. Feel all of your tension dissolving into the water. Your body feels lighter, like you are floating.

Take a deep abdominal breath. Smile into your heart and then into every area of your body. Imagine golden light flowing into your head and face, into your neck and shoulders, into your arms and hands, into your chest and back, into your abdomen and waist, into your hips and thighs, into your knees and lower legs, and into your feet. Feel your body tingling with energy. You are calm and peaceful. This is just one example. Be creative and imagine the desired outcome as if it has already happened.

Let me tell you one story of how I used visualization in my own life. I had developed a condition called hyperthyroidism (thyroid is overactive), where my metabolism was greatly increased. This caused my resting heart rate to increase to an extreme point, more than one hundred beats per minute (way too high).

I was so uncomfortable and it was difficult for me to relax. I would use a pulse oximeter to measure my heart rate throughout each day. I knew that a good average resting heart rate was around 60 beats per minute (bpm), so I would sit down with my eyes closed and visualize that my pulse oximeter was showing 60 bpm, even though it really said 100 bpm. I also did abdominal breathing while visualizing.

While I did see a doctor, I chose not to take medication. I chose a more natural approach to deal with this issue including adjusting my nutrition and supplementation. And total elimination of stress. After about three weeks of daily visualizations (many times throughout the day), my resting heart rate came down.

It eventually returned to around 65 bpm. This is only an illustration and is not a substitute for proper medical treatment. If you have a health condition, see your doctor immediately. Then in conjunction with the doctor's treatment, you can employ these techniques to aid in your healing.

While you are visualizing, it is best to do abdominal breathing. This will enhance your relaxation. If you've been stressed out for some time, it will take consistent practice to reverse the physical effects of stress. But it can be done.

Visualize how you will be and what it will feel like when you have accomplished your goal of relaxation or whatever it is that you want to accomplish. Imagine that you have already achieved your desired outcome or the end result. Dr. Wayne Dyer called it "Thinking from the end."

If you want to make your visualizations even more effective, then practice your visualizations five minutes or so before going to bed. This will place positive, empowering thoughts in your mind that will then be processed by your subconscious mind during sleep. Not only that but it will put you in a relaxed state that is conducive to going to sleep.

This is very important if you have difficulty sleeping at night because your mind is racing. Now you have a very powerful tool to focus your mind with positive and empowering thoughts that will relax you and put you in the right mind for sleeping. If you wake up in the middle of the night and find it difficult to go back to sleep, what do you do? Visualize and breathe. Just imagine the possibilities.

Here's another hint. Visualization is not only good for just relaxing, you can use it for any situation or result that you would like to achieve. Practice it regularly and you will relax your mind and achieve your desired outcome. Practice. Practice. Practice.

Action Steps

It is now time for you to put visualization into practice in your life. Sit in a comfortable and quiet place. Close your eyes and visualize yourself in a situation that is calming and relaxing. What does it look like? How does it feel? What do you smell? Try to involve as many of your five senses as possible.

Continue to visualize in this way for five minutes or longer. Now express your gratitude for this time and your experience. When you are done, take out your journal and write down your visualization and what you noticed and experienced. You can repeat this visualization daily to create change in your life. Be patient. Practice daily and have fun with it.

CHAPTER 8 – RETURN TO NATURE

"The Doctor of the Future will give no medicine, but will involve the patient in the proper use of food, fresh air, and exercise."
- Thomas Edison

When was the last time you took a walk in nature? We get so caught up in our complex daily lives that we sometimes forget about the simple joys of life. For me, walking in the park is one of those simple joys that I look forward to occasionally. I realize that it is difficult to just let go of our responsibilities and enjoy the simple things in life. Or is it?

As I have said previously, we do what we choose to do. I hope that you have learned by now that you can make a choice to take some time for yourself. Consider it like self-maintenance or preventative maintenance.

Why not choose to relax before you are forced to because your blood pressure is too high? Why not choose to relax before you have an anxiety attack? Why not choose to relax before you get to the point where you cannot shutdown your mind and go to sleep? In case you haven't noticed, you have a choice. Walking in nature is a choice that I make, as often as I can. It is one of my favorite preventative maintenance techniques.

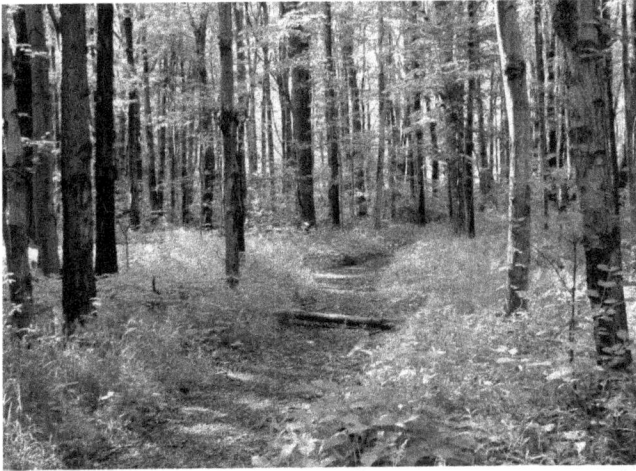

I find that being in the *"here and now"* in nature is one of the most peaceful and relaxing things I can do. I like to walk on a nature trail and just observe nature. I will make a fun game of it. I will see how many different living things I can observe. This may include birds, geese, ducks, turtles, frogs, ants, dragonflies, fish, deer, trees, and flowers or more on any given day.

Just observing nature helps us to realize that we humans are part of a very large family of living beings on planet Earth. We are truly connected and dependent on every living being. When we let go of our worries and just be present with the mysteries of life itself, which is especially evident in nature, it can be not only freeing to our mind, but it can also be healing to our mind and body. Walking in nature is truly a moving meditation.

I have to warn you to not consider your walk in nature as an extension of the office. For the purpose of relaxation, you should turn your cell phone and other gadgets off while you are walking in nature. I can't tell you how many times I see several people walking together and one of them is on the cell phone. They are not being present with the person or child they came with. I also see people walking with their headphones on listening to the ball game or music.

While there is a time and a place for these things, they are not appropriate on the relaxation walk in nature that I am referring to. I want you to walk and let go of everything else for at least a half-hour, though longer is better.

Here's a simple practice that you can do in nature. Sit down on a bench, a chair, or the grass in the park and close your eyes. Take a deep breath. Listen to the various sounds in nature. What do you hear? Nature sounds differently when we close our eyes because our minds are no longer distracted and we hear things we hadn't really paid much attention to before.

Can you hear the birds singing? Can you hear the leaves rustling in the wind? Can you hear the geese honking? Can you hear the water trickling down the stream? Can you hear the crickets chirping? It's amazing what you can hear when you close your eyes. Just listen and breathe. That is enough to calm a busy mind.

Action Steps

It is time to take action. Schedule time to walk in the park, even if it is cold outside with snow on the ground. Take a walk in nature and just be in the moment. Do abdominal breathing as you are walking. Put a smile on your face. Notice the things around you. What do you see? What do you hear? What do you feel?

If you find your mind wandering, just acknowledge that it is wandering and return your thoughts to your surroundings in nature and to your breathing. Do not judge your thoughts. Do not resist your thoughts. Just return your mind to the *"Here and Now"*, the present moment.

After your walk, write down in your journal how you felt during your walk. Write down what you noticed about being in the present moment during your walk. Was it easy? Did you feel connected to nature? Write down anything that comes to mind.

CHAPTER 9 – TEN MINUTE RELAXATION MEDITATION

"I hear and I forget; I see and I remember; I do and I understand."
- Chinese Proverb

At this point, you have learned many individual meditation techniques to use on a daily basis. Now let's put it all together into a simple ten minute meditation program that can be done daily. And we will even throw in some body relaxation. After all, we are holistic beings with a mind and body.

Keep in mind that throughout your day, when you can't sit down for a regular meditation, that you can still use the meditation techniques in this book individually. Read this chapter first before starting your meditation practice, so you learn and understand the basic structure of the meditation and so you can take time to prepare for the meditation.

Setting your intention for the meditation practice is very important. First, you must prepare for the meditation, including setting your intention. Then you can practice the meditation.

Prepare Yourself for Meditation

1. Find a quiet and comfortable place where you won't be interrupted. Turn off your cell phone and other distractions.
2. It is best to sit up in a chair so you won't be tempted to go to sleep. If you do fall asleep don't worry, it happens. You can either return to your meditation or try again later when you feel more awake.
3. Sit up with your back straight and your feet flat on the floor. Don't cross your legs because this will restrict blood flow and energy to your legs. You can either fold your hands on your lap or put your hands palm down on your thighs.
4. Close your eyes, take a deep breath, and let it out slowly.
5. Put a smile on your face.
6. Set your intention for the meditation.
   I choose to

   _____

   _____.

   Fill in the blank. For example: relieve stress, forgive someone, feel more relaxed, feel more joy, ... etc.

   Now come up with a simple positive affirmation that represents your desired outcome.

   Here's several examples:

I am calm, peaceful, and relaxed.
I am able to go to sleep on time.
I can quiet my mind whenever I choose to.

Begin Meditation (10 minutes)

1. Repeat Your Affirmation (1 minute)

Repeat your affirmation internally over and over for a minimum of one minute. Focus on the words. This will help you to focus your mind.

2. Be in the "Here and Now" (1-2 minutes)

Just sit and witness what you are thinking and feeling without any judgments. Don't try to dismiss them or resist them. That will only give them more energy.

By just noticing your thoughts without resistance, they will eventually go away on their own. Then another thought will come up. Keep witnessing your thoughts and feelings for a minute or two.

3. Abdominal Breathing (2 minutes)

Do abdominal breathing for several minutes. Inhale slowly, gently and deeply into your abdomen. Exhale slowly, gently and deeply.

You can count your breath cycles. Inhale, exhale, 1. Inhale, exhale 2. Inhale, exhale 3. Keep doing abdominal breathing and counting your breath for 2 minutes. You will find it relaxing and refreshing.

Remember the keys to effective abdominal breathing are: **slow, long, thin, even and soft**.

4. Visualization (2 minutes)
Now visualize achieving the outcome that you set with your intention and affirmation. Involve as many of the five senses as you can for the best results. Don't forget to do abdominal breathing (don't count, just breathe).

For example, if your intention was to feel relaxed, then you could visualize yourself sitting on a beach. Feel the warm ocean breeze on your face. See the bright sunshine. Hear the waves gently splashing on the beach.

Reach down and take a handful of sand and let it pour down to the ground. Hear the sounds of the seagulls flying overhead. It is a tropical paradise. Put a smile on your face. Feel relaxed and comfortable. Say your affirmation (quietly) as you listen to soothing sounds of the ocean. I am relaxed.

5. Relax Your Body (2 minutes)
Now relax each part of your body starting with your head and gradually moving down towards your toes. Start with your head. Put your attention on your face

and head. Imagine all tension releasing from your face and head.

If you find it difficult to relax your face and head, you can lightly tense your head and face. Then release the tension. Feel the tension melting away.

Repeat this for your neck, shoulders, arms, hands, chest, back, abdomen, pelvis, legs, and feet. You can spend extra time in areas that do not release. Once you reach your feet, repeat the entire process again.

6. Finish Your Meditation (1 minute or less)

Now we can finish this meditation with a statement of gratitude. Express silently to yourself whatever you are thankful for. Be truthful and honest. It can be about the meditation or about anything else in your life. For example: I am grateful for experiencing relaxation during this meditation.

Now slowly open your eyes and notice how you are feeling. If you want, you can write in your journal about your experience and how you feel after.

The most important thing about meditation is practice. Practice daily for the best results. Don't worry about doing each step perfectly. Just do something to start and you will get better at it. With practice, it will get easier and the benefits will increase. Have fun with it. And to make it better, invite a friend or family member to join you.

Action Steps

Before practicing this meditation program, take out your journal and write down your intention for your practice. Then come up with a positive affirmation that represents your intention and write it down.

Now you can start with the preparation section and proceed into practicing the meditation. Once you have completed your practice for at least ten minutes, write your experiences down in your journal. How did the meditation feel? Were you able visualize yourself achieving your desired outcome? Also write down what you are grateful for.

CHAPTER 10 – CONCLUSION

"The path to success is to take massive, determined actions."
\- Tony Robbins

In the previous chapters, you learned what stress is and how it manifests in your mind and body. You learned that the root cause of stress is fear. And now you know what it means to *"relax your mind"*; letting go of the mindless, subconscious chatter, brought about by negative programming from fear-based stressful perceptions.

You learned that when you practice being in the present moment, the *"Here and Now"*, you can let go of your perceptions and judgments about the past and future and just be.

You learned meditation techniques for transforming your mind from chaos to relaxation, through *"silent witnessing"*, positive affirmations and mantras, focusing your mind, calming your mind, and retraining your mind.

You learned how to **retrain your subconscious mind** with conscious thoughts and choices, which can help to change, manage, or eliminate fears and stress. It was also presented that forgiveness and gratitude were key to relaxing the mind.

You also learned how to do **abdominal breathing**. You learned about the many benefits that comes with abdominal breathing, including increased oxygen and energy, increased circulation, lower blood pressure, massaging the internal organs, and of course relaxation.

By now, I hope you have been practicing these meditation techniques to relax your mind. If you have, then you know first-hand how simple, but powerful, the techniques are for relaxing your mind. As stated previously, the benefits are numerous and life changing. While it does take time to practice the techniques, the benefits are worth it in the long run.

The long list of potential benefits include, relaxing the mind, stress relief, lowered blood pressure and heart rate, improved immune function, improved digestion, improved blood circulation, improved energy, improved mental focus and concentration, healthier lifestyle, and so on.

Don't take my word for it. Continue practicing these meditation techniques and see how they change your life in two weeks, in six weeks, in three months, in six months, in one year, in two years, in five years and so on.

Keep writing your experiences in your journal. If you find yourself going down a stressful path, review your journal and know that you can steer yourself back on the path.

Our conscious mind can be both our most powerful asset and our worst adversary. It is our choices that define who we are and what we can accomplish. When we make empowering conscious choices and stay rooted in the present moment, we create a powerful and beneficial asset. And when our thoughts are ruled by our negatively programmed subconscious mind, we create an adversary, which sabotages our thoughts and actions.

So now it is up to you to make a choice between stress and relaxation. You have all the tools you need to choose relaxation. I hope you choose to **relax your mind**.

From The Author

First of all, thank you for purchasing this book "*Relax Your Mind.*" I know you could have picked any number of books to read, but you picked this book and for that I am extremely grateful.

I hope that it added value and quality to your everyday life. If so, it would be really nice if you could share this book with your friends and family by posting to **Facebook** and **Twitter**.

If you enjoyed this book and found some benefit in reading this, I'd like to hear from you and hope that you could take some time to post a review on Amazon. Your feedback and support will help this author to greatly improve his writing craft for future projects and make this book even better.

You can follow the link to **Relax Your Mind** now at https://www.amazon.com/dp/B07H1PMN62.

Your review is very important and so, if you'd like to leave a review, all you have to do is click **here**, https://www.amazon.com/dp/B07H1PMN62, and it will take you to the book page.

If you'd like to get notifications of new book releases, special offers, and other related content, please join my email list at
https://www.EliminateStressNow.com/esn-join-our-email-list/

I wish you all the best in your future success!

REFERENCES

1. *"Nomophobia"*, Wikipedia.org. Web Retrieved December 30, 2015 from https://en.wikipedia.org/wiki/Nomophobia.

2. Walia, Arjun. (2014, December 11). *"Harvard Study Unveils What Meditation Literally Does To The Brain"*, Collective-Evolution.com. Web Retrieved January 2, 2016 from http://www.collective-evolution.com/2014/12/11/harvard-study-unveils-what-meditation-literally-does-to-the-brain.

3. *"Meditation for Anxiety"*, Headspace.com. Web Retrieved January 2, 2016 from https://www.headspace.com/science/meditation-for-anxiety.

4. Moyer, Melinda Wenner. (2014, May 1). *"Is Meditation Overrated?"* Scientific American. Web Retrieved January 2, 2016 from http://www.scientificamerican.com/article/is-meditation-overrated.

5. Black, David S., et. al. (2015, April). *"Mindfulness Meditation and Improvement in Sleep Quality and Daytime Impairment Among Older Adults With Sleep*

Disturbances" The JAMA Network. Web Retrieved January 2, 2016 from http://archinte.jamanetwork.com/article.aspx? articleid=2110998.

6. *"America's #1 Health Problem"*, "The American Institute of Stress. Web Retrieved January 8, 2016 from http://www.stress.org/americas-1-health-problem.

7. *"Stress (biology)"*, Wikipedia.org. Web Retrieved January 8, 2016 from https://en.wikipedia.org/wiki/Stress_(biology).

8. *"The Relaxation Response"*, Wikipedia.org. Web Retrieved January 8, 2016 from https://en.wikipedia.org/wiki/The_Relaxation_Response

9. Go, Jowett. *"Transforming Your Negative Self-Talk as your Inner Coach – A 4 Step Approach"*, The Performance Institute. Web Retrieved January 3, 2016 from http://www.theperformanceinstitute.com.au/transforming-negative-self-talk-inner-coach-4-step-approach.

10. Page, Sam. *"How to Rewire Your Brain: The Science Behind Affirmations"*. Sam Page Fitness. Web Retrieved January 3, 2016 from http://www.peacelovelunges.com/topics/health/get-rid-of-fear-and-pain-once-and-for-allpgsxmyifiuhtvhqa2piwq.

11. *"Using Affirmations Harnessing Positive Thinking"*, MindTools. Web Retrieved January 3, 2016 from https://www.mindtools.com/pages/article/affirmation s.htm.

12. *"Respiratory system"*, Wikipedia.org. Web Retrieved January 8, 2016 from http://en.wikipedia.org/wiki/Respiratory_system.

ABOUT THE AUTHOR

Thomas Calabris has studied and practiced various forms of meditation and Qigong for almost thirty years. He studied meditation, Qigong, and Tai Chi from Grandmaster Robert Krueger. Most recently, he studied Inner Dan Arts Qigong (meditation and exercise) with Grandmaster Tianyou Hao, since January 2001. Thomas is a certified instructor of Inner Dan Arts Qigong. He also studied Qinway Qigong with Grandmaster Qinyin and Wisdom Healing Qigong with Master Mingtong Gu. He holds a Bachelor of Science Degree in Electrical Engineering and a Master of Science Degree in Biomedical Engineering. He currently develops software as a software engineer. He has also studied anatomy and physiology and various areas of natural health. He brings a unique perspective of science, tradition, and experience to his teachings.

Learn more about stress relief at:
http://www.EliminateStressNow.com

Learn more about Qigong at:
http://www.InnerVitalityQigong.com

Ten Minute Relaxation Meditation Checklist

Preparation
1. Find a quiet place to practice.
2. Sit up in a chair with your back straight.
   Feet flat on the floor.
3. Fold hands on your lap or put palms down on
   your thighs.
4. Close your eyes, take a deep breath, and let it
   out.
5. Put a smile on your face.
6. Set your intention for the meditation.

Meditation
1. Repeat your affirmation (1 minute)
2. Be in the "Here and Now", silent witnessing
   (1-2 minutes)
3. Abdominal Breathing (2 minutes)
4. Visualize your desired outcome (2 minutes)
5. Relax Your Body (2 minutes)
6. Finish your meditation with gratitude
   (1 minute or less)

BOOKS BY THE AUTHOR

Relax Your Mind: Simple Meditation Techniques to Relieve Stress and Quiet a Busy Mind

Learn more at:
https://www.amazon.com/dp/B07H1PMN62

Relax Your Mind Companion Workbook: A Guide To Learn Meditation Techniques to Relieve Stress and Quiet a Busy Mind

Learn more at:
https://www.amazon.com/dp/B07YRWVZSJ

Healing Stress: Effective Solutions for Relieving Stress and Living a Stress-Free Life

Learn more at:
https://www.amazon.com/dp/B07KVNXN14

The Color of Relaxation: Adult Coloring Book for Stress Relief and Relaxation

Learn more at:
https://www.amazon.com/gp/product/1086248295

Dreams Into Reality: Manifest Your Dreams Into Being Using The Law Of Attraction

Learn more at:
https://www.amazon.com/dp/B081NVJ94G